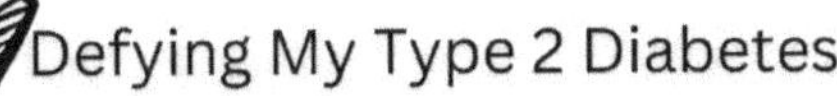

HOW A REGULAR PERSON RECLAIMED HIS HEALTH AND YOU CAN TOO!

James S. Andersen

DEFYING MY TYPE 2 DIABETES

How a Regular Person Reclaimed His Health and You Can Too!

James S. Andersen

Enlightened 2.0 Publishing

CONTENTS

INTRODUCTION

(OR, WHY ARE WE HERE)

Hi there, my name is James and I'm just a regular guy - a computer programmer from New York with a wife, three kids, two cats, and even a parakeet. You know, the kind of guy who's constantly juggling the demands of career, family, and all the other responsibilities that seem to define modern life.

As someone who spends a lot of time staring at lines of code, I tend to approach problems with a very analytical, data-driven mindset. So just four years ago, when I was hit with a type 2 diabetes diagnosis at the young age of 35 - you can bet I didn't just accept it and resign myself to a lifetime of medications and restrictions.

Instead, I saw it as a challenge to be studied, decoded, and systematically conquered. Just like debugging a complex software issue, I was determined to leave no stone unturned in my quest to regain control of my health. And let me tell you, the transformation I was able to achieve through that process has been nothing short of life-changing.

<u>Let me start with a disclaimer</u>: I am not a doctor, dietitian, or any kind of credentialed medical expert. I'm just a regular family guy who was fortunate enough to discover a path to reversing my own type 2 diabetes diagnosis through dedicated research and lifestyle modifications. This is solely my personal journey, and the information in this book should not be taken as medical advice as it may be inaccurate, misleading or even utterly wrong for you, especially if you have a medical history, clinical state or a pregnant woman.

This book is my personal story, and the information within should not be taken as medical advice. Your individual needs and circumstances may be vastly different from mine. What worked for me may or may not work perfectly for you. But I firmly believe that the principles and strategies I've learned can serve as a powerful blueprint for taking control of your health destiny, no matter how bleak your current situation may seem.

Before making any changes to your diet, exercise routine, or medication regimen, it is absolutely crucial that you consult your healthcare provider. Your doctor knows your unique medical history and needs best, and should be an integral part of your diabetes management plan. I cannot and will not tell you to stop taking your prescribed medications or to ignore your physician's guidance. That would be both irresponsible and potentially dangerous.

That said, I firmly believe the principles and strategies I've learned can serve as a powerful blueprint for taking control of your health destiny, no matter how bleak your current situation may seem. And I'm going to share them with you in the most transparent, relatable way I know how - through the lens of my own experience as a regular person just like you.

You see, when I first heard those dreaded words, "you have type 2 diabetes," my mind immediately swirled with visions of being slowly crippled by this chronic disease, missing out on watching my kids grow up, and becoming yet another dismal statistic in the ever-growing diabetes epidemic. I was filled with a sense of dread, uncertainty, and utter hopelessness.

But then something inside me shifted. I refused to accept that narrative. I refused to be medicated before I explored all of my options. While I tremendously respect the medical profession and believe consulting with your doctor is wise when embarking on any health journey, I also came to realize that many physicians simply don't have all the answers when it comes to managing conditions like diabetes. Their conventional treatment protocols too often revolve around just managing symptoms through medications and one-size-fits-all dietary guidelines, rather than actually getting to the root cause of the issue.

At the end of the day, no one knows your body better than you. As human beings, we're imbued with incredible innate healing potential if we just take the time to listen to our intuition and tap into lifestyle choices that are truly in alignment with our biological needs. This realization was a pivotal turning point for me.

Faced with the grim prognosis of my type 2 diabetes diagnosis, I refused to go down without an all-out fight. I was determined to take my health into my own hands using holistic, natural, and sustainable methods - no matter how daunting the challenge might seem. Little did I know then just how transformative that decision would prove to be.

By tapping into the latest scientific research and studying the real-life experiences of people who had beaten their diabetes diagnoses, I soon discovered a roadmap back to health and vitality that I never thought was possible. Yes, it took overhauling my nutrition, exercise, sleep, and stress management practices from the ground up. But doing so allowed me to completely reverse my diabetes in a matter of months - Through my systematic, data-driven approach - much like the way I tackle complex programming challenges , I was able to completely overhaul my nutrition, fitness, sleep, and stress management habits. And in just the first 4 months, I lost 30 pounds and reversed my diabetes diagnosis entirely (!!!), ditching the thought of taking medications for good.

If you too find yourself staring down diabetes or another daunting health crisis, I have good news: You hold the power to rewrite your story. With the right knowledge, tools, mindset shifts, and self-belief, you can kick diabetes squarely in the rear and reclaim your wellness. And in the pages ahead, I'll guide you through the exact steps I took to do just that.

You see, as a computer programmer, I'm no stranger to tackling complex challenges through a systematic, data-driven approach. And that's precisely the mindset I brought to my diabetes diagnosis. I was determined to leave no stone unturned in my quest for answers, drawing insights from the latest scientific research as well as the real-life experiences of those who had beaten the condition.

Just like debugging a tricky software issue, I meticulously tracked my biometrics, experimented with different interventions, and continuously refined my approach based on the data. It wasn't always a linear process, and there were certainly plenty of ups and downs along the way. But by staying curious, flexible, and committed to the end goal, I was able to systematically dismantle the root causes of my insulin resistance and reclaim my health.

Throughout the pages ahead, I'll share the nutrition, fitness, sleep, and stress management hacks that allowed me to reverse my type 2 diabetes diagnosis. I'll also dive deep into the mindset shifts and self-care practices that kept me resilient and motivated, even in the face of setbacks. And I'll emphasize the vital importance of personalization, self-discovery, and trusting your own intuition as you navigate this transformative journey. For your convenience, each chapter holds a "Tips, Hacks, and Takeaways" section where you can find the main points I want you to concentrate – exactly like I did.

My hope is that by sharing my experiences - the triumphs and the challenges, the breakthroughs and the learning moments - I can inspire you to take that first step towards reclaiming your health. Because I know from firsthand experience that the power to overcome even the most daunting of diagnoses lies within you. You just have to be willing to claim it.

So if you're ready to embark on this life-changing expedition, know that you don't have to go it alone. I'll be with you every step of the way, drawing from my own experiences to guide you through the inevitable obstacles and victories that lie ahead.

In these pages, I'll guide you through the exact lifestyle changes I made that allowed me to do just that. You'll discover delicious, nutrient-dense recipes, creative workout tips, and a treasure trove of holistic, natural health hacks that made the path to wellness not just possible, but incredibly rewarding.

No more restricting and feeling deprived. No more grueling two-hour daily grind sessions. Just a simple, sustainable blueprint for optimizing your body's own healing powers - while still enjoying an abundantly flavorful life!

By the time you reach the end of this book, my hope is that you'll not only have a comprehensive blueprint for reversing your type 2 diabetes, but you'll also possess the unshakable belief, resilience, and self-knowledge to keep that reversal permanent. No more settling for just managing your condition - it's time to take back your health and wellness for good.

You've got this. I know because I was once in your shoes, and diabetes no longer has a hold over me. Now it's your turn to become the boss of your own biology!

Are you ready to take your power back? Then let's dive in and get started!

1. UNDERSTANDING DIABETES

Diabetes is a serious health condition that affects how your body manages and uses sugar (glucose) for energy. When you have diabetes, your body either doesn't produce enough of the hormone insulin, or it can't use the insulin it does produce effectively. This leads to high levels of glucose building up in your bloodstream instead of being properly absorbed by your cells.

There are two main types of diabetes:

Type 1 Diabetes: This is an autoimmune condition where your body mistakenly attacks and destroys the insulin-producing cells in your pancreas. It's usually diagnosed at a younger age and requires insulin injections to survive.

Type 2 Diabetes: This is the more common form of diabetes, and the one I personally struggled with. It's closely linked to lifestyle factors like poor diet, lack of exercise, and chronic stress. In type 2 diabetes, your cells become resistant to the effects of insulin, so your body can't regulate blood sugar levels properly.

For me, the road to type 2 diabetes started with

some unhealthy habits that had crept into my life over the years. As a busy, working dad, I often found myself grabbing quick, processed meals on the go instead of nourishing my body with whole, unprocessed foods. The constant flow of refined carbs, added sugars, and unhealthy fats from these convenient but nutrient-poor foods quietly eroded my metabolic health.

On top of that, I was routinely skimping on sleep and letting stress accumulate unchecked. Late nights spent working long hours at the office left me chronically fatigued, my delicate hormonal balance thrown completely out of whack. On a cellular level, the combination of poor nutrition, lack of rest, and unmanaged stress was creating the perfect storm for insulin resistance to develop.

On its own, any one of these lifestyle factors can increase your risk of type 2 diabetes. But when they pile up - poor diet, sedentary behavior, sleep deprivation, and constant stress - it becomes a veritable recipe for metabolic disaster. The glucose and insulin regulation systems that normally keep your blood sugar in a healthy range start to malfunction, leading to that dreaded type 2 diabetes diagnosis.

And the consequences of uncontrolled diabetes can be truly devastating. Chronically high blood sugar levels put strain on your blood vessels, nerves, and organs, leading to serious complications like nerve damage, vision loss, kidney disease, and even cardiovascular events. It's no wonder that so many people with diabetes live in fear of these life-altering consequences.

But here's the good news: you have the power to take control of this condition and potentially even reverse it. By making strategic, sustainable changes to your nutrition, fitness, sleep, and stress management habits, you can restore balance to your body's metabolic processes and reclaim your health. It won't be easy, but I'm living proof that it's absolutely possible.

In the chapters ahead, I'll walk you through the exact steps I took to completely turn my type 2 diabetes around. You'll discover science-backed strategies for optimizing your diet, igniting your metabolism through the right exercise routines, and cultivating the mindset shifts that allowed me to overcome this diagnosis for good.

The road may have its fair share of ups and downs, but I promise you this: by the time you reach the end of this book, you'll be armed with the knowledge, tools, and unshakable belief that you can rewrite your health destiny. Diabetes no longer has to be the boss of you. It's time to take your power back.

Are you ready? Then let's dive in and get started!

💡 Tips, Hacks, and Takeaways

- Recognize that lifestyle factors like poor diet, lack of exercise, chronic stress, and sleep deprivation are the primary drivers of type 2 diabetes development.

- Understand that the consequences of uncontrolled diabetes - nerve damage, vision loss, kidney disease, and cardiovascular issues - can be truly devastating if left unchecked.

- Get motivated by the fact that type 2 diabetes is reversible through strategic, sustainable changes to your nutrition, fitness, sleep, and stress management habits.

- Commit to becoming an empowered, proactive partner in your own health journey, rather than passively relying on medications or generic advice from "experts."

- Maintain unwavering hope and belief that you can rewrite your health destiny, no matter how bleak your current circumstances may seem.

2. SMASHING DIABETES MYTHS & MISCONCEPTIONS

As you embark on this journey of reversing your diabetes through nutrition and lifestyle adjustments, there's no doubt you'll encounter plenty of skeptics and naysayers. From well-meaning friends and family, to even some medical professionals doubting your ability to ditch medications or escape the diagnosis altogether, you're bound to get an earful of misconceptions along the way.

In this chapter, we'll be debunking some of the most common diabetes myths while sharing a treasure trove of hard-truth tips and tricks for lasting success. Consider this your tough-love pep talk to overcome any lingering self-doubt or disbelief that you can absolutely take control of your health destiny!

Myth #1: Diabetes is a chronic, progressive disease that can't be reversed

Distinguishing between type 1 and type 2 diabetes is critical here. For those with an autoimmune condition where their body attacks and destroys insulin-producing cells, that form of diabetes isn't currently reversible through lifestyle alone. Type 2 diabetes, however, is a metabolic condition largely driven by dietary and lifestyle factors like excess weight, lack of exercise, poor sleep, and other stressors. By removing the root causes, you can most certainly regain normal blood sugar control!

I'm living proof of this. When I was first diagnosed with type 2 diabetes at the age of 35, my doctor painted a bleak picture of a chronic, progressive condition that would only worsen over time. But by overhauling my nutrition, ramping up my fitness regimen, and optimizing my sleep and stress management, I was able to completely reverse my diabetes in a matter of months - no more endless medications, painful injections, or compromise of quality of life.

The latest research backs up my experience, with numerous studies demonstrating that comprehensive lifestyle interventions can lead to full diabetes remission in a significant percentage of patients. It may take dedication and persistence, but the scientific evidence is clear: type 2 diabetes is a reversible metabolic disorder, not an irreversible life sentence.

Myth #2: You'll be miserable deprived of carbs and sweets

While limiting your intake of refined carbs and sugars is advisable for optimizing insulin sensitivity, think of it more as upgrading your fuel sources rather than deprivation. There are still plenty of amazing, flavorful dishes incorporating healthy fats, lean proteins, low-glycemic veggies, fruits, nuts, and seeds that will leave you satisfied - no hangriness required! Not to mention keto-friendly desserts that allow you to indulge smarter.

In fact, one of the biggest surprises for me on my diabetes reversal journey was just how delicious and satisfying this way of eating can be. Rather than feeling deprived, I found myself expanding my culinary horizons and discovering a whole new world of nutrient-dense ingredients that energized and satisfied me in a way processed, sugary foods never could.

From rich, fudgy chocolate brownies made with coconut flour to crispy baked zucchini fries dipped in creamy cashew "ranch", I was able to still enjoy plenty of comforting, crave-worthy treats - I just had to get a bit more creative in the kitchen. And you know what? I found that with a little experimentation, these diabetes-friendly dishes often tasted even better than the junky versions I used to indulge in.

The key is to approach this dietary shift with an open mind and a spirit of curiosity, rather than seeing it as a rigid set of rules. Tune out the naysayers who insist you'll be miserable and deprived, and instead focus on all the amazing, flavorful possibilities that await you. Your taste buds (and your waistline) will thank you.

Myth #3: You have to exercise for hours a day to reverse diabetes

More is not better when it comes to fitness for diabetes. In fact, excessive cardio could end up reinforcing insulin resistance if not fueled strategically. Instead, focus on shorter bouts of strength training, HIIT, and low-intensity movement. Anything getting you breathless for under an hour is plenty to enhance insulin sensitivity long-term.

I used to think that I had to be spending hours upon hours in the gym, pushing myself to the brink of exhaustion, in order to overcome my type 2 diabetes. But I quickly learned that this approach wasn't just unsustainable - it was actually counterproductive. The intense stress and metabolic demands of endless cardio sessions ended up elevating my cortisol levels and further undermining my insulin sensitivity.

What worked infinitely better were targeted,

strategic workouts that revved my metabolism, depleted my glycogen stores, and built up my lean muscle mass - all in just 30-60 minutes a few times per week. Things like full-body strength training, high-intensity interval training (HIIT), and brisk daily walks had a much more profound, lasting impact on my glucose control than grinding away for hours on the treadmill.

The key is to find movement that you genuinely enjoy and can realistically fit into your lifestyle on a consistent basis. It doesn't have to be complicated or extreme - in fact, the simpler and more sustainable, the better. The goal is to keep your body challenged and engaged, not to punish or deprive yourself.

Myth #4: Diabetes medications are the only reliable solution

When it comes to type 2 diabetes, the conventional medical approach often heavily relies on a pharmaceutical intervention model. Doctors will typically prescribe metformin, insulin, or a combination of diabetes drugs as the frontline treatment, with the assumption that these medications are the only reliable way to manage blood sugar levels.

However, what this mindset fails to account for is the root cause nature of type 2 diabetes and the incredible power of lifestyle modification to fundamentally shift the underlying metabolic dysfunction. While medications can certainly be a useful temporary crutch, they do not address the dietary, activity, stress, and sleep habits that originally sparked the insulin resistance process.

In fact, an over-reliance on drugs can sometimes backfire, masking the need for deeper lifestyle changes and potentially leading to worsening of the condition over time as the body becomes further desensitized to insulin. The better approach is to view medications as a short-term tool, while simultaneously implementing the sustainable dietary, fitness, and stress management practices that can put you on the path to complete diabetes reversal.

I'm not suggesting you should ever abruptly stop taking your prescribed medications without first consulting your doctor. That would be extremely unwise and potentially dangerous. What I am saying, however, is that you have the power to work collaboratively with your healthcare provider to gradually wean off those drugs as your body regains its metabolic balance. With the right holistic interventions, many individuals are able to achieve normoglycemia and diabetes remission without the need for endless prescriptions.

Myth #5: Diabetes is your genetic destiny

Finally, it's important to address the pervasive myth that type 2 diabetes is simply an inescapable genetic fate - that if it runs in your family, you're doomed to develop the condition no matter what you do. While family history and certain genetic predispositions can certainly increase your risk, they do not condemn you to a life of poor health.

The human genome is incredibly complex, with countless variables that influence disease risk. But what the latest research makes abundantly clear is that lifestyle factors - particularly diet, physical activity, stress management, and sleep quality - play a massively outsized role in determining whether those genetic susceptibilities ever actually manifest.

In other words, your genes are not your destiny when it comes to type 2 diabetes. Even if you have a strong family history of the condition, you possess the power to modify your environmental triggers and epigenetic expression to dramatically reduce your chances of developing it. With the right knowledge and commitment to sustainable lifestyle changes, you can absolutely overcome the odds stacked against you.

I'm living proof of this. When I was first diagnosed with type 2 diabetes at a relatively young age, my doctor assumed it was simply my genetic fate, given my family history. But by taking an active, empowered role in transforming my nutrition, fitness, sleep, and stress management habits, I was able to completely reverse the diagnosis in a matter of months - no medications required.

So as you embark on this journey of diabetes reversal, I encourage you to let go of any lingering fears, doubts, or preconceived notions you may have about the condition. Dismiss the naysayers, ignore the diabetes management "experts" touting costly drugs and rigid restrictions, and instead focus your energy on becoming an empowered student of your own unique biology.

Your body possesses an incredible capacity for self-healing - you just need to create the right conditions for it to thrive. And that, my friend, is precisely what the rest of this book is all about. So are you ready to start rewriting your health destiny? Then let's dive in!

💡 Tips, Hacks, and Takeaways

- Reject the notion that type 2 diabetes is a chronic, irreversible condition. It is reversible through comprehensive lifestyle changes.
- Ignore claims that a low-carb, high-fat diet is deprivation. It's about upgrading your

fuel sources, not sacrificing flavor and satisfaction.

- Disregard the myth that endless hours of grueling exercise are required. Strategic, moderate workouts are far more effective.
- Understand that medications are not the only solution. You can work collaboratively with your doctor to gradually wean off them.
- Dismiss the idea that your genes doom you to diabetes. Lifestyle factors have a much greater impact on disease risk.
- Approach this journey with unwavering self-belief and an empowered mindset, not self-doubt or resignation.

3. MASTERING YOUR METRICS

Before making any major changes to your diet, exercise routine, or medication regimen, there's one absolutely crucial step you must take: start closely tracking and analyzing your blood glucose levels.

Think of it like a meteorologist studying weather patterns - you need accurate data about what's really going on inside your body in order to understand how your daily choices and lifestyle factors are impacting your diabetes. Only then can you make informed, strategic decisions to get your blood sugar under control.

Now, I know what you might be thinking - constantly pricking your finger to check your glucose is a hassle you'd rather not deal with. But I'm here to tell you that game-changing continuous glucose monitors (CGMs) have made the whole process smoother and more insightful than ever before.

CGMs use a tiny sensor inserted just under your skin to track your glucose levels 24/7, syncing the data to your smartphone or a separate receiver. This means you can get real-time updates on your blood sugar without ever having to draw another drop of blood. You can also install an additional no cost app to show the history of several days back and more importantly during the night.

Instead of sporadic, scattered finger prick measurements, you'll have a constant, comprehensive window into how your body is responding to everything from the foods you eat to your exercise sessions and stress levels. The ability to see these patterns unfold in real-time is truly transformative.

For example, you might notice that a breakfast of oatmeal and fruit causes a massive blood sugar spike, while a protein-rich scramble keeps your levels nice and stable. Or you could discover that taking a brisk 30-minute walk after lunch has a much more profound impact on lowering your post-meal glucose than an hour-long cardio session. I did, those discoveries made all the difference for me.

The beauty of this continuous glucose monitoring is that it allows you to become a true biohacking expert on your own body. Rather than relying on generic dietary advice or one-size-fits-all exercise routines, you can start to uncover the personalized strategies that work best for regulating your unique metabolism.

Beyond just observing your glucose patterns, pairing your CGM data with periodic testing of your blood ketone levels can also provide invaluable insights. When your body is in a state of nutritional ketosis - where fat and ketones become your primary fuel source rather than glucose - it can have a profound positive impact on insulin sensitivity, oxidative stress, and overall metabolic health.

Incorporating targeted fasting protocols, like intermittent or extended fasts, can be a highly effective way to shift your body into this fat-burning, ketosis state. And by tracking your glucose and ketone levels with your CGM, you can fine-tune these fasting regimens to find what works best for your unique biology.

Of course, embarking on any fasting program, especially if you're currently taking diabetes medications, should always be done under the guidance of your healthcare provider. But with the right support and precautions, periodic fasting can be an incredibly powerful tool in your diabetes-conquering arsenal.

Beyond just glucose and ketone monitoring, continuously tracking other key biomarkers like HbA1c, cholesterol, blood pressure, and inflammation levels can also yield invaluable big-picture insights about your overall metabolic health. This allows you to proactively address any potential imbalances before they spiral into full-blown complications.

I know that the world of biohacking and self-quantification can feel overwhelming at first. But I encourage you to approach it with a spirit of curiosity and enthusiasm, not dread. This is your opportunity to become an empowered citizen scientist, taking an active, data-driven role in your own healthcare. Think of it as an investment in your most precious asset - your health and vitality.

With the right tools and a little practice, this level of deep self-knowledge will transform the way you approach managing your diabetes. No more guessing, no more frustrating trial-and-error. You'll have a "glucose crystal ball" that reveals exactly how your body responds to different foods, activities, and lifestyle factors in real-time.

Imagine the freedom and confidence that comes with that kind of self-mastery! No more fears of "falling off the wagon" due to an unexpected blood sugar spike. Instead, you'll be equipped with the data and insights to course-correct in the moment, then quickly get back on track.

So what are you waiting for? It's time to start hacking your blood sugar and taking your health into your own hands! Invest in a high-quality continuous glucose monitor, download a user-friendly app to track your data, and get ready to embark on a fascinating journey of self-discovery. Your diabetes-reversing superpowers await!

💡 Tips, Hacks, and Takeaways:

- Invest in a high-quality continuous glucose monitor (CGM) to get real-time, 24/7 insights into your body's glucose regulation. Don't forget the accompanying apps for long term history measures.

- Use your CGM data to become a biohacking expert on your own unique metabolism, identifying the specific foods, activities, and lifestyle factors that impact your blood sugar.

- Pair your glucose monitoring with periodic testing of blood ketone levels to optimize your body's ability to efficiently burn fat for fuel.

- Work closely with your healthcare provider when incorporating fasting protocols, as dramatic shifts in blood sugar can be dangerous without proper medical guidance.

- View the process of self-quantification and biomarker tracking as an empowering investment in your health, not a burdensome chore.

4. DIABETES-CRUSHING DIET

If you were to sum up the core philosophy of diabetes reversal in just a few words, it would be: "Let food be thy medicine, and medicine be thy food." At its essence, type 2 diabetes is rooted in insulin resistance, where your body's cells stop responding properly to the insulin your pancreas produces to regulate blood sugar. The key, therefore, is to give your body's hormones and signaling processes a "reset" by limiting the influx of glucose and getting sugar levels under control.

When it comes to reversing type 2 diabetes, your diet is undoubtedly one of the most powerful levers you have at your disposal. After all, the foods you choose to fuel your body with play a direct and profound role in regulating your blood sugar, insulin sensitivity, and overall metabolic function.

That's why the very first step in my own diabetes reversal journey was overhauling my nutrition - swapping out the refined carbs, added sugars, and inflammatory processed foods that were silently eroding my health for a diet centered around nutrient-dense, blood sugar-stabilizing whole foods.

Now, I know what you might be thinking - "But

James, does that mean I have to give up all my favorite foods and go on some super restrictive diet?" Absolutely not! In fact, one of the key lessons I learned is that achieving lasting diabetes control isn't about deprivation at all. It's about upgrading the quality and composition of the foods you consume.

You see, the dietary approach that worked wonders for me, and that I believe can be truly transformative for anyone looking to get their type 2 diabetes under control, is a low-carb, moderate protein, high healthy fat way of eating. This is sometimes referred to as a "keto" or "paleo" style of nutrition, but the specific labels don't really matter. What's important is the principles behind it.

By limiting your intake of quickly-digested, blood sugar-spiking carbohydrates - like breads, pastas, rice, potatoes, and sugary treats - and instead emphasizing foods that are rich in fiber, healthy fats, and slow-burning complex carbs, you can systematically dial down the inflammation and insulin resistance that are at the root of type 2 diabetes.

Think leafy greens, avocados, olive oil, nuts and seeds, lean proteins like salmon and chicken, and low-glycemic fruits and veggies. These nutrient-dense ingredients not only help stabilize your blood sugar, but also provide lasting satiety and steady, high-octane energy that leaves you feeling satisfied, not sluggish and deprived.

And the best part is, with a little creativity in the kitchen, you can still enjoy all sorts of crave-worthy, diabetes-friendly meals and treats. Instead of reaching for refined flour and sugar, I've found amazing substitutes like almond flour, monk fruit sweetener, and nut-based "cheese" sauces that allow me to indulge in things like decadent brownies, crispy baked "fries," and creamy, savory casseroles.

Cutting out sugary drinks like soda and juice has also been a game-changer for me. I used to be a big fan of adding spoonfuls of sugar to my coffee and tea, but now I've trained my taste buds to appreciate the natural flavors without any sweeteners.

It was tough at first, but after just a week or two, I no longer craved those sweet, blood sugar-spiking beverages. When it's hard, I drink zero sugar drinks or chew zero sugar gum and it does the trick. Myths about the damages it can cause in terms of progress diabetes, are just myths as far as I can tell for the past four years.

The same goes for all the carb-heavy foods I used to rely on, like bread, pasta, and potatoes. In the beginning, it felt like a real sacrifice to give them up. But as my body adapted to burning fat and ketones for fuel instead of glucose, those cravings started to fade. Now I genuinely enjoy the satisfying, nourishing meals I prepare, without ever feeling deprived.

Of course, transitioning to this style of eating will require some adjustments, both in the kitchen and in your mindset. Gone are the days of mindlessly reaching for processed, convenience foods. Instead, you'll be learning to read labels, experiment with new recipes, and tune in to the unique ways your body responds to different foods.

But trust me, it's a small price to pay for the incredible benefits you'll reap. As you start to experience the transformative effects of stabilizing your blood sugar - increased energy, clearer focus, reduced inflammation, and even potential weight loss - you'll realize that this isn't deprivation at all. It's liberation.

The key is to approach this dietary shift with curiosity, self-compassion, and an open mind. Rather than seeing it as a rigid set of rules, view it as an opportunity to explore, experiment, and truly tune in to what your body thrives on. With a little creativity and the right mindset, you might just be surprised by how delicious and satisfying this "diabetes-friendly" way of eating can be.

Of course, you'll need to work closely with your healthcare provider to ensure any dietary or medication changes are implemented safely. And remember, there's no one-size-fits-all solution - what works perfectly for me may not necessarily be the optimal approach for you. The beauty is in the process of personalized discovery.

So are you ready to dive in and start dialing in your diabetes-crushing diet? Let's get started!

💡 Tips, Hacks, and Takeaways:

- Use high-quality sugar substitutes like monk fruit or stevia to satisfy sweet cravings without spiking your blood sugar.
- Experiment with alternative flours like almond, coconut, or cassava to make keto-friendly baked goods and breads.
- Load up on healthy fats from sources like avocados, olive oil, nuts, and seeds to stay satisfied between meals.
- Increase your intake of protein-rich foods like meat, poultry, eggs, and cheese to help regulate blood sugar.
- Eliminate sugary drinks like soda, juice, and sweetened coffee/tea, which can rapidly elevate glucose levels.
- Expect an adjustment period, but know that

after about a week, your body and taste buds will start to adapt to the new way of eating.

- Focus on progress, not perfection. Small, sustainable steps in the right direction will lead to powerful, lasting transformation.

5. WORK OUT SMARTER, NOT HARDER

While dialing in your diet is undoubtedly the foundation for reversing type 2 diabetes, it's only one piece of the puzzle. The other crucial component is finding the right exercise strategies to support your metabolic transformation.

Now, I know what you might be thinking - "But James, I thought diabetes was all about watching what I eat. Do I really need to be slaving away at the gym for hours on end too?" The answer is a resounding yes...and no.

You see, when it comes to fitness for diabetes, the old notion that "more is better" couldn't be further from the truth. In fact, I found that lengthy, grueling workout sessions often ended up doing more harm than good, elevating my stress levels and exacerbating insulin resistance.

What worked infinitely better for me were targeted, strategic routines that combined three key elements:

1) Strength training to build lean muscle mass and boost my metabolic rate

2) High-intensity interval training (HIIT) to rapidly deplete glycogen stores and enhance insulin signaling

3) Low-intensity movement to ensure I was consistently burning fat for fuel

Let me break down each of these components and explain why they've been so game-changing for my diabetes reversal efforts.

Strength Training for Metabolic Firepower

When it comes to reversing insulin resistance, building and maintaining lean muscle mass has been one of the single most important factors for me. Muscle tissue is a metabolically active organ that plays a crucial role in glucose uptake and utilization - the more I have, the more efficiently my body can clear sugar from my bloodstream and shuttle it into my cells for energy.

Interestingly, the very biochemical processes that become impaired in insulin resistance - like glucose transporter expression and insulin receptor function - can actually be upregulated and optimized through targeted resistance training. It's like giving my body's glucose regulation systems a complete tune-up.

Now, I used to think that I needed to be pumping

iron like a bodybuilder to reap these metabolic benefits. But research has actually shown that low-to-moderate load resistance training with higher repetitions can be just as effective, if not more so, for enhancing insulin sensitivity in individuals with type 2 diabetes.

The key for me has been to focus on compound, multi-joint exercises that recruit large muscle groups, like squats, deadlifts, pull-ups, and pushups. These types of movements stimulate a powerful hormonal cascade, including the release of growth hormone and testosterone, that supports my metabolic rate, body composition, and glucose control.

I try to incorporate 2-3 full-body strength sessions per week, keeping each workout relatively brief (30-45 minutes) but high in intensity. And I've found that doing these sessions in the morning, shortly after a protein-rich breakfast, allows my muscles to efficiently utilize the incoming nutrients as fuel.

High-Intensity Interval Training (HIIT) for Glycogen Depletion

Alongside my strength training efforts, high-intensity interval exercise has been another crucial component of my diabetes-conquering fitness regimen. HIIT workouts, which involve short bursts of maximal-effort exercise followed by periods of active recovery, have been a game-changer for improving my insulin sensitivity and glucose control.

The reason these types of workouts are so beneficial has to do with the way they rapidly deplete the glycogen stores in my muscles and liver. This glycogen-depleting effect, in turn, signals my body to become more efficient at clearing glucose from my bloodstream and utilizing it for energy, rather than storing it as fat.

Beyond just the glycogen-depleting benefits, HIIT has also been shown to enhance the expression and translocation of glucose transporters like GLUT4 to the cell membrane. This allows more glucose to be taken up by my muscle cells, rather than remaining in circulation and contributing to hyperglycemia.

And the cherry on top? These intense, anaerobic workouts also stimulate the release of fat-burning hormones like growth hormone and catecholamines. They even elevate my metabolic rate for hours after a session, helping me continue to burn calories and fat even when I'm at rest.

I try to fit in a HIIT workout a few times per week, usually in the afternoon a couple hours after my lunch. This allows my body to have fully digested and utilized the nutrients from the meal, while also taking advantage of the natural dip in cortisol that occurs in the mid-to-late afternoon.

And you know what? I don't need to spend hours upon hours doing these intense bursts of exercise to see remarkable results. In fact, just 10-20 minutes a few times per week has been incredibly impactful for me. Something as simple as 30-second sprints followed by 90 seconds of active recovery can be a highly effective diabetes-busting routine.

Low-Intensity Movement for Sustained Fat-Burning

While the resistance training and HIIT workouts have been essential pillars of my fitness routine, I've also found that incorporating plenty of low-intensity movement has been crucial for enhancing my insulin sensitivity and promoting fat loss - two key factors in my diabetes reversal journey.

The reason low-intensity exercise has been so beneficial has to do with the way our bodies utilize different fuel sources. During higher-intensity workouts that deplete my glycogen stores, I primarily burn carbohydrates for energy. But during lower-intensity, steady-state activities, I shift towards burning stored body fat as my primary fuel source.

This fat-burning effect has been particularly advantageous for me, as excess abdominal fat was a major contributor to the development and progression of my type 2 diabetes in the first place. By regularly engaging in low-intensity movement like brisk walking, leisurely hiking, and easy swimming, I've been able to steadily chip away at that stubborn fat, while also improving my body's ability to clear glucose from my bloodstream.

In terms of timing, I've found that the best time for my low-intensity workouts is first thing in the morning, before I've eaten breakfast. By going for a brisk walk or doing some light yoga in a fasted state, I'm able to tap into my body's fat-burning pathways and further enhance my insulin sensitivity throughout the day.

An added benefit is that these low-intensity workouts are generally less taxing on my body than the high-intensity intervals or heavy strength training sessions. This has made them an ideal option for days when I'm feeling fatigued, sore, or simply need an active recovery session. I can still reap tremendous diabetes-fighting benefits without risking burnout or overtraining.

So what does a balanced, diabetes-conquering fitness routine look like for me in practice? Here's a sample weekly plan I've been following:

Monday: 20 mins HIIT (cycling between max effort sprints and active recovery) - Afternoon

Tuesday: Full-body resistance workout using my own bodyweight or light weights - Morning

Wednesday: 45-60 minute brisk walk outdoors - Morning

Thursday: Repeat Monday's HIIT session - Afternoon

Friday: Repeat Tuesday's resistance training - Morning

Saturday: Rest and recover

Sunday: Gentle yoga or light cardio if desired - Afternoon

Of course, I started slow when I first began this fitness journey, gradually building up the duration, intensity, and variety of my workouts over time. But the key things I've focused on are: a) getting my heart rate up and then allowing it to drop back down, b) lifting weights that challenge me but don't overtax my muscles, and c) consistently incorporating low-intensity movement like walking to coax my body into burning fat for fuel.

The goal hasn't been to work myself into the ground, but rather to strategically challenge my body in ways that enhance my insulin sensitivity, glucose control, and fat-burning. Moderation, progression, and self-awareness have been crucial - not grueling, endless workouts.

As I've experimented with different workout styles and found what resonates most with my unique physiology, I've started to notice some incredibly powerful, tangible benefits. I've experienced better energy levels, improved sleep quality, reduced inflammation, and even some weight loss - all of which have further supported my efforts to conquer type 2 diabetes for good.

But the fitness piece of the puzzle isn't just about the physical act of moving my body. The mental and emotional components have played a huge role as well. Cultivating a joyful, empowered mindset around exercise - versus seeing it as a dreaded chore - has made all the difference in my ability to stick with it long-term.

I've found ways to make my workouts fun, social, and intrinsically motivating, whether that's trying new activities, exercising outdoors in nature, or working out alongside supportive friends and family members. The more I can infuse my fitness routine with a sense of play, discovery, and personal growth, the more sustainable and diabetes-busting it's been.

So if you're ready to start revving your metabolism and taking your diabetes reversal efforts to the next level, I'm here to tell you that it's entirely possible. Grab your sneakers, get creative, and let's get moving together!

💡 Tips, Hacks, and Takeaways:

- Incorporate targeted resistance training 2-3 times per week to build lean muscle mass and boost your metabolic rate.
- Focus on compound, multi-joint exercises that recruit large muscle groups, like squats, deadlifts, pull-ups, and pushups.
- Try high-intensity interval training (HIIT) a few times weekly to rapidly deplete glycogen stores and enhance insulin sensitivity.
- Prioritize low-intensity movement like brisk walking, hiking, or easy swimming to promote fat-burning and further improve glucose control.
- Time your workouts strategically, doing strength training in the morning and HIIT in the afternoon for optimal results.
- Start slow and gradually increase the duration, intensity, and variety of your fitness routine over time.
- Cultivate a joyful, empowered mindset

around exercise by finding activities you genuinely enjoy and making them a social experience.

6. MASTERING STRESS & SLEEP

While meticulously watching your nutrition and fitness habits are critical pieces of the diabetes reversal puzzle, they'll only get you so far if you're not also attending to two often-overlooked pillars of optimal health: stress management and sleep quality.

You see, study after study has shown strong links between insufficient sleep, elevated stress hormones like cortisol, and increased insulin resistance/risk for type 2 diabetes. When your body remains in a constant state of perceived threat - whether from work deadlines, relationship tensions, or even just a restless night's sleep - it hoards glucose and energy for potential "fight-or-flight" scenarios. This chronic stress response blunts your cells' ability to properly utilize insulin, leading to persistently high blood sugar levels.

That's why, in addition to overhauling my diet and exercise routine, prioritizing high-quality sleep and implementing effective stress management practices have been absolutely vital to my own success in reversing type 2 diabetes. These often-overlooked lifestyle factors have played just as crucial a role, if not more so, than any single dietary or fitness strategy.

Let's start with sleep. When it comes to optimal rest and recovery, it's not just about logging a certain number of hours under the covers - it's also crucially important to ensure you're cycling through the various sleep stages, from light to deep to REM, in the appropriate amounts and timing. This allows your body and brain to engage in the vital restorative processes that support metabolic health, immune function, cognitive performance, and so much more.

One of the best ways to optimize this sleep architecture is by regulating your exposure to light, both natural and artificial. Our bodies are highly sensitive to light cues, which act as the primary zeitgebers (time-givers) for our circadian rhythms. By minimizing blue-wavelength light exposure in the evenings and getting ample natural daylight during the day, you can help synchronize your body's internal clock for more efficient, high-quality sleep.

Beyond just the quantity and quality of your slumber, the final piece of the sleep puzzle is ensuring your sleeping environment is optimized for maximal rest and recovery. Things like temperature, noise, and even the mattress and pillow you use can dramatically impact your ability to fall and stay asleep. Experiment with adjustments until you find the conditions that allow you to truly drift off and wake feeling refreshed.

Now, I know what you may be thinking - "But James, I'm a busy parent/professional/caretaker...how on earth am I supposed to get 7-9 hours of sleep per night?" I hear you, and I completely understand the challenges of prioritizing shut-eye in our fast-paced world. That's why it's so crucial to get creative and make sleep optimization a non-negotiable part of your daily routine.

For me, that has meant things like adjusting my work schedule to allow for an earlier bedtime, outsourcing household tasks, and even enacting a "digital sunset" where all screens are powered down two hours before I want to be asleep. It's also meant leaning on my support system - whether that's my partner, family members, or even a sleep coach - to hold me accountable and remind me of the life-changing benefits of high-quality rest.

The dividends of prioritizing your sleep are absolutely immense, especially when it comes to reversing insulin resistance and conquering type 2 diabetes. By ensuring you're cycling through the various sleep stages and maintaining healthy circadian rhythms, you'll be supporting everything from glucose regulation and fat metabolism to immune function and mood stability.

What's more, the stress-reducing effects of quality sleep can have a profound impact on your ability to manage diabetes-related challenges with resilience and equanimity. When your mind and body are well-rested, you're far better equipped to navigate the ups and downs, maintain motivation, and keep your eye on the big picture of long-term wellness.

Of course, effective stress management is the other crucial piece of the mind-body puzzle. As I mentioned earlier, ongoing psychological and physiological stress can have a tremendously detrimental impact on insulin sensitivity and glucose regulation. When your body perceives threats, whether real or imagined, it responds by pumping out hormones like cortisol that raise blood sugar to provide quick energy for potential "fight-or-flight" scenarios.

The problem is, in our modern world of constant digital distractions, work deadlines, relationship troubles, and other daily stressors, this stress response often stays activated for far too long. Chronically elevated cortisol can blunt insulin's effects, causing blood sugar to remain stubbornly high even when insulin is present.

Beyond just the direct metabolic consequences,

excessive stress can also wreak havoc on your mental and emotional well-being - two other vital components of successful diabetes reversal. When you're perpetually anxious, depleted, and overwhelmed, it becomes exponentially harder to maintain the motivation, focus, and self-compassion required to make the necessary lifestyle changes.

So what's the solution? Well, just like with sleep, it all comes down to establishing consistent, sustainable stress management practices that help regulate your mind-body responses. For me, that has meant incorporating a diverse toolkit of techniques, from breathwork and meditation to journaling and leisure activities.

One of my go-to practices is the 4-7-8 breath pattern, which has been shown to have a powerful calming effect on the nervous system:

1) Breathe in through your nose to a count of 4

2) Hold that breath inside for a count of 7

3) Slowly release the breath through pursed lips to a count of 8

Just a few rounds of this simple breathing exercise can trigger your parasympathetic ("rest and digest") nervous system responses, counteracting the detrimental impacts of stress hormones. I'm always amazed at how much more centered and resilient I feel after taking a few minutes to focus on my breath.

Another daily ritual that's been incredibly valuable is my morning journaling practice. I'll spend 10-15 minutes free-writing about any swirling thoughts, fears, or frustrations causing me angst. Getting that mental clutter out of my head and onto paper is like taking out the trash - it creates spaciousness for me to then write down affirmations and set positive intentions for the day ahead.

I've also found great benefit in incorporating more leisure activities and "playtime" into my routine, whether that's reading fiction, going for leisurely hikes, or trying new creative hobbies. Actively carving out space for enjoyment, wonder, and self-expression has been crucial for managing stress and avoiding burnout on this wellness journey.

Of course, the specific stress management techniques that work best for you may look quite different from mine. The key is to experiment and find a diverse toolkit of practices that resonate with your unique personality, lifestyle, and needs. The more variety you can build in, the better equipped you'll be to handle the inevitable ups and downs.

Ultimately, the goal is to cultivate a lifestyle of holistic mind-body harmony - one where you're giving your nervous system the consistent cues it needs to shift out of that chronic "fight-or-flight" state and into a state of calm, restorative rest and digest. When you can do that, the positive impacts on your metabolic health, energy levels, and quality of life will be truly profound.

So as you continue your journey of diabetes reversal, I encourage you to approach the sleep and stress management pieces with the same commitment and creativity you're bringing to your diet and fitness regimens. These often-overlooked lifestyle factors are absolutely vital to the bigger picture of reclaiming your vitality.

Remember, you're not just fighting to control your blood sugar - you're fighting to restore balance, resilience, and joy to every aspect of your being. And with the right holistic strategies in place, I have full confidence that you can not only conquer type 2 diabetes, but emerge as the happiest, healthiest version of yourself. Let's do this!

💡 **Tips, Hacks, and Takeaways:**

- Prioritize 7-9 hours of high-quality sleep

per night by optimizing your sleep environment and regulating your exposure to light or noise.

- Implement effective stress management practices like breathwork, meditation, journaling, and leisure activities to counteract the detrimental effects of chronic stress.
- View sleep and stress management as essential, non-negotiable components of your diabetes reversal efforts, not optional add-ons.
- Get creative and enlist the support of your loved ones to help you overcome barriers to prioritizing rest and relaxation.
- Remember that your physical and mental wellbeing are inextricably linked - optimizing both is key for reversing insulin resistance and reclaiming your vitality.

7. EMBRACING THE UPS & DOWNS

Even armed with all the right knowledge of nutrition, exercise, sleep, and stress management, the road to diabetes reversal is rarely a straight shot. Inevitably, you'll deal with motivation lapses, "cheat day" overindulgences, schedule snafus, and other setbacks along the way that make it tempting to throw in the towel.

This is exactly why developing a mindset of supreme grit, resilience, and self-compassion is so vital. More so than any single diet, workout, or piece of technology, your ability to learn from temporary failures, shake them off, and get back on track is what will ultimately make or break your success.

So on those days when the brownie craving gets the best of you or you just don't have the oomph for a home HIIT workout after a crazy workday, don't beat yourself up! Pause, reset your intentions, and treat it like training for your mental toughness muscle.

Here are some strategies that can help you swiftly move past stumbling blocks:

• Reflect and journal about what prompted the slip-up. Was it stress, boredom, fatigue? Get curious about it without judgment.

• Make a specific plan for getting right back into your routine, no matter how small. Even just a walk outside can shift your energy.

• Celebrate all wins, no matter how tiny! Meeting your daily hydration goal? Smashed it! Hit your step count target? You're a rockstar!

• Call in support from others who can encourage and uplift you. Share your progress and struggles for accountability.

• Visualize yourself already at your healthy, thriving best. How does that version of you act? What habits does that person have?

Embracing setbacks not as failures, but inevitable minor obstacles to power through, is what will see you shattering through plateaus again and again. Just remember - resilience is what separates those who talk about making changes from the ones who actually manifest lasting results.

The Power of Pivoting, Not Perfection

One of the biggest mental hurdles I've had to overcome on my diabetes reversal journey has been letting go of the notion of perfection. For so long, I put immense pressure on myself to get everything "just right" - my meals had to be 100% on point, my workouts had to be grueling, and my sleep and stress management had to be flawless.

But the reality is, life doesn't work that way. There will always be unexpected challenges, curveballs, and moments of weakness that derail even the most disciplined efforts. And beating myself up over those "failures" only served to further undermine my confidence and momentum.

What I've learned is that true, sustainable progress comes not from perfection, but from the power of pivoting. It's about having the grit and self-compassion to quickly course-correct when things go awry, without getting mired in shame or self-doubt.

For example, let's say I had planned to meal prep a week's worth of keto-friendly lunches over the weekend, but life got in the way and I didn't have time. Rather than throwing my hands up and resigning myself to a week of fast food, I might instead pivot to keeping some simple go-to items on hand, like pre-cooked chicken, bagged salads, and easy veggie sides. It's not the elaborate plan I had envisioned, but it's better than abandoning my efforts entirely.

Or what if I wake up one morning and just don't

have the energy or motivation for my usual HIIT workout? Instead of berating myself, I could pivot to a gentler, lower-intensity activity like a brisk walk or some light yoga. The key is to avoid the all-or-nothing mentality and remember that any movement is better than no movement.

The same principle applies to my nutrition. If I find myself craving a sweet treat in a moment of stress or boredom, I don't have to see that as a catastrophic "failure" that ruins my whole day. I can simply pivot to one of my pre-planned "emergency" options, like a square of dark chocolate or a small portion of berries with whipped cream. A minor indulgence, not a free-for-all.

The beauty of this pivoting mindset is that it allows me to maintain consistency and momentum, even when life throws me curveballs. Rather than beating myself up over every little slip-up, I can acknowledge it, learn from it, and quickly get back on track. It's about progress, not perfection.

Of course, that's easier said than done, especially when you're first starting out on this journey and old habits and thought patterns feel so ingrained. That's why it's so crucial to also cultivate unwavering self-compassion as you navigate the ups and downs.

Whenever I find myself slipping into the trap of harsh self-judgment, I try to stop and ask myself: "Would I talk to a dear friend this way if they were in my shoes?" The answer is almost always a resounding "no." We tend to be so much harder on ourselves than we would ever be on someone we care about.

So I make a conscious effort to respond to my own setbacks and stumbles with the same kindness, empathy, and encouragement I would offer a loved one. I remind myself that slip-ups are inevitable, and that the true mark of success lies not in perfection, but in the ability to bounce back quickly with renewed determination.

Sometimes, that might mean taking a day or two to truly rest and recharge, free from any self-imposed demands. Other times, it means leaning on my support system of friends and family who can remind me of how far I've come and cheer me on. And often, it's simply a matter of pausing, taking a few deep breaths, and reflecting on the progress I've already made.

The key is to shift my mindset away from criticizing and berating myself, and towards approaching each challenge as an opportunity for growth. How can I learn from this setback? What can I do differently next time? What small, sustainable step can I take right now to get back on track?

By cultivating that spirit of curiosity, flexibility, and self-compassion, I've found that the inevitable ups and downs of this journey become much easier to navigate. The failures and plateaus don't derail me - they simply become part of the process, temporary obstacles to power through on my way to long-term transformation.

Where Do You Want to Be in a Year?

Of course, embracing setbacks and maintaining resilience is only half the battle. The other crucial piece is keeping your eye firmly fixed on the big-picture vision of the healthy, thriving future you want to create.

It's all too easy, when you're in the thick of the daily grind, to lose sight of that end goal and get mired in the minutiae of meal planning, workout schedules, and data tracking. But I've found that regularly reconnecting with that deeper sense of "why" - the powerful motivation that first sparked your desire for change - can be the difference-maker in powering through tough times.

For me, that bigger "why" is the vision of being fully present and engaged with my wife and kids, brimming with natural energy and vitality, for many years to come. I don't want to just survive - I want to truly thrive. I want to be there for all of life's milestone moments, doing cartwheels in the front yard rather than sitting on the sidelines, weighed down by the debilitating effects of uncontrolled diabetes.

When I find myself struggling with motivation or feeling tempted to give in to old habits, I'll often take a few moments to vividly imagine that future version of myself. What does my day-to-day life look like? How do I move, think, and feel? What activities and experiences am I able to freely enjoy? By tapping into that positive mental imagery, I'm able to reconnect with the profound importance of the work I'm doing in the present.

I also find it incredibly helpful to create tangible reminders of that desired future state - whether it's vision boards, affirmations, or even just placing meaningful photos around my home and workspace. Surrounding myself with visual cues of the healthy, vibrant life I'm working towards keeps me motivated and inspired, even on the most challenging days.

Additionally, I make it a point to regularly celebrate the small wins and incremental progress I make along the way. Rather than only ever focusing on the big, distant goal of "curing" my diabetes, I make a conscious effort to acknowledge and feel proud of each milestone, no matter how tiny.

Maybe it's finally breaking through a weight loss plateau, or nailing a new strength training PR, or simply maintaining a stable blood sugar range for an entire week. Whatever it is, I make sure to take a moment to acknowledge it, reflect on how far I've come, and let that sense of accomplishment fuel my continued forward momentum.

Of course, it's not always easy to maintain that positive, big-picture perspective, especially when you're feeling discouraged or defeated. That's why it's so crucial to have a strong support system in place - whether that's loved ones, a diabetes-focused community, or even a professional coach or therapist.

Sharing your progress, challenges, and ultimate vision with others who can provide encouragement, accountability, and fresh perspectives can be an absolute game-changer. There have been countless times when a conversation with a friend or a pep talk from my spouse has been the lifeline I needed to get unstuck and regain my determination.

Ultimately, the key is to approach this journey of diabetes reversal with an unwavering commitment to self-compassion, flexibility, and long-term thinking. Setbacks and stumbles are inevitable, but with the right mindset and strategies in place, you can turn them into powerful opportunities for growth, rather than allowing them to derail your efforts.

Remember, you're not just fighting to control your blood sugar - you're fighting to reclaim your vibrant health, your quality of life, and your ability to fully show up for the people and experiences that matter most to you. And with grit, resilience, and a clear vision of your desired future, I have every confidence that you can and will achieve that ambitious, life-changing goal.

Where do you want to be one year from today? Sitting on the couch, shackled by another health crisis? Or out living your best life, stamina through the roof, doing cartwheels with your loved ones? The choice, my friend, is yours to make. So let's get to work!

💡 Tips, Hacks, and Takeaways:

- Approach setbacks and slip-ups with curiosity and self-compassion, not harsh self-judgment.
- Develop strategies for quickly pivoting and

getting back on track, even if it's just a small, sustainable step.

- Celebrate every win, no matter how minor, to stay motivated and focused on your progress.
- Lean on your support system of friends, family, and healthcare providers to provide encouragement and accountability.
- Maintain a clear, inspiring vision of your desired healthy, thriving future to power you through challenging times.
- Remember that perfection is not required - consistent effort and self-compassion are the keys to lasting transformation.

8. CONCLUSION: RECLAIMING YOUR HEALTH DESTINY

As I put down the pen on recounting my experience, reflecting on my journey brings a huge smile to my face. I'm overjoyed to have taken my health back into my own hands through the power of lifestyle and determination. It's been a life-changing transformation that has restored my energy, my freedom, and my ability to fully show up for the people and experiences that matter most to me.

If you're reading this and have also been diagnosed with type 2 diabetes - or are fighting any other kind of health issue - please know that you have the power to change your circumstances too. I know it may seem daunting, even impossible, in the face of a grim prognosis or the seemingly endless medications, restrictions, and compromises that come with a chronic condition. But I'm here to tell you that it is absolutely possible to reclaim your vitality and thrive.

Of course, it will take real effort, discipline, and commitment to shifting your ingrained habits around food, exercise, sleep and managing stress. Transforming your metabolic health isn't something that happens overnight, nor is it a linear process free of setbacks and challenges. But as you've seen through my story, the rewards of persevering through those difficulties can be truly life-changing and extraordinary.

Never lose hope or succumb to doom and gloom thinking. You can beat this! Whether you apply the exact tactics I've shared here or find your own personalized path, I encourage you to keep exploring, remain curious about new solutions, and most importantly - believe in yourself. Listen to that inner voice that tells you you're stronger than your struggles.

Throughout this book, I've aimed to provide you with a comprehensive, evidence-based blueprint for taking control of your health destiny. I've shared the nutrition strategies, fitness routines, sleep hygiene practices, and stress management techniques that allowed me to completely reverse my type 2 diabetes diagnosis. And I've emphasized the vital importance of self-compassion, resilience, and a long-term, big-picture mindset in navigating the inevitable ups and downs of this journey.

But at the end of the day, this is your journey. No one can do the work for you. The power to rewrite your health story lies firmly within your grasp - you just have to be willing to claim it. So I urge you, with every fiber of my being, to take that first step. Reach out to your healthcare provider, invest in a continuous glucose monitor, and start experimenting with lifestyle changes that move the needle for your unique biology.

It's been such an honor to share my experiences in hopes of inspiring your own healing transformation. From the bottom of my heart, I wish you unwavering courage and the best of luck as you write the next chapters of reclaiming your health and happiness!

The road ahead may have its share of hills and valleys, but I have every confidence that you possess the grit, resilience, and self-belief to emerge victorious. Diabetes no longer has to be the boss of you. It's time to take your power back and become the architect of your most vibrant future.

So what are you waiting for? The first step is always the hardest, but I promise you, it gets easier with each passing day. Gather your support system, clear your schedule for some much-needed self-care, and dive headfirst into this transformative journey. Your body, your mind, and your loved ones are counting on you.

The time is now. The power is yours. Let's do this!

9. BONUS CHAPTER 1: GROCERY & KITCHEN HACKS

While the nutrition principles for reversing type 2 diabetes are simple in theory - limit refined carbs, eat plenty of fiber, focus on healthy fats and proteins - putting them into practice in the real world can seem infinitely more complicated.

From decoding nutritional labels and identifying hidden sugar traps, to battling cravings while grocery shopping, to meal prepping flavorful diabetes-friendly dishes, successfully overhauling your dietary habits requires strategic planning and know-how.

In this chapter, I'll be sharing my own hard-won wisdom and favorite tips for optimizing your kitchen set-up and grocery routines. These insights will empower you to create a home environment that nudges you towards sustainable, blood sugar-stabilizing food choices, while still allowing you to enjoy immensely satisfying, craveable meals.

Let's start at the supermarket, where one of the biggest pitfalls is being lured in by deceptive food marketing and sneaky added sugars. You know logically that the bakery section and inner aisles lined with processed snacks aren't going to do your metabolic health any favors. But grocery stores are carefully designed environments that leverage music, lighting, strategic product placing, and even aroma piping to trigger cravings and impulse purchases.

My number one tip? Stick to the perimeter of the store for the most part. That's where you'll find the fresh produce, meat/seafood, dairy, bulk bins for nuts/seeds, and other whole, minimally-processed ingredients. Only venture into the inner aisles for a few key staples like:

-Oils like olive, avocado & coconut

-Condiments like mustard, hot sauce, apple cider vinegar

-Canned fish (look for kinds packed in water)

-Spices & dried herbs

-Unsweetened nut butters

Speaking of nut butters, one of the biggest mistakes I see is people who have been intimidated by overly-restrictive low-fat diets and constant calorie counting. I used to fear nuts, nut butters, olive oil, and other healthy fats, assuming they'd derail my progress. But these nutrient-dense foods are absolutely crucial for providing lasting satiety, stable energy levels, and supporting nutrient absorption.

So make sure your grocery cart is loaded with them - everything from crunchy almonds and pecans to creamy almond butter and fresh avocados. Just be mindful of portion control.

When it comes to selecting your proteins, feel free to mix it up with a variety of poultry, eggs, seafood, red meat, and even plant-based options like tofu and tempeh. But be extremely wary of pre-made, processed meats like deli slices, sausages and fish products that tend to be loaded with sodium, preservatives, and hidden sugars.

As for the produce section, God's candy aisle as I affectionately call it, load up! You simply cannot go wrong by filling your cart with leafy greens, cruciferous veggies, ripe avocados, nutrient-dense berries, etc. But you'll want to learn the difference between high and low-glycemic fruits so you're balancing things properly. Pro tip: Frozen fruits and veggies can be just as nutritious as fresh, and infinitely more convenient.

To up-level your grocery haul, consider looking

for a local ethnic grocery store. These gems often have unique produce varieties, harder-to-find ingredients, and generally much lower prices than chain supermarkets. I've discovered some of my favorite keto swaps and cooking staples this way.

For pre-packaged snacks and foods, arm yourself with knowledge by diligently reading nutrition labels. Look for items that are low in net carbs (subtract fiber from total carbs) and have minimal added sugars. Beware of ingredients like maltodextrin, dextrose, brown rice syrup, concentrated fruit juices and fiberless flour blends - these sneaky sugars can spike insulin levels.

If you find yourself tempted by less-than-optimal items at the store, pause and ask yourself - is this worth potentially derailing my progress and feeling out of control around food again? Often that thought exercise is enough for me to stay disciplined.

And one last grocery shopping hack - never go to the store while ravenously hungry! Always try to fuel up on a protein-rich snack or shake before venturing out to avoid impulsive, regrettable purchases.

Now let's talk setting up your kitchen for diabetes-friendly success! Here are my must-have tools and strategies for meal prep:

Invest in a high-quality chef's knife, cutting boards, basic pots/pans, baking sheets, food storage containers, small kitchen scale for measuring portions, and a sturdy blender or food processor. Having the right equipment makes healthy eating infinitely easier.

I also highly recommend picking up a few kitchen gadgets like a veggie spiralizer for making nutrient-dense noodle alternatives, an Instant Pot for effortless meal prep, and a mandoline for quick veggie slicing. Not strictly necessary, but incredible time-savers.

Clear off a section of countertop space dedicated solely to food prep, and keep it clutter-free. Having a clean workspace with tools readily accessible removes friction from the cooking process.

Spend a few hours weekly prepping ingredients ahead of time - whipping up a batch of protein balls, hard boiling eggs, pre-chopping veggies, pre-portioning nuts and energy bites. It makes healthy snacking and meal assembly a total breeze.

Create a stash of portable, diabetes-friendly meal

preps that you can grab and go for days you don't have time to cook. Think lettuce wraps, pre-made salads with protein/healthy fats, or little snack boxes filled with crunchy veggies, nuts, and olives.

If dining out, try to scout the menu ahead of time and go in with a game plan, whether that's ordering a bunless burger nestled in a lettuce wrap or asking to sub in extra veggies for high-carb sides. Restaurant meals can easily derail your hard work, so preparation is key.

Finally, be patient and kind with yourself as you adapt to new shopping and cooking routines! It can feel overwhelming at first, but with some practice, it will become second nature - no more time than you likely spent on your former less-than-optimal dietary habits.

Tap into your support network when you need a pep talk or could use a hand in the kitchen. And try out new recipes and meal prep hacks to keep things fun, interesting and sustainable in the long run.

Ultimately, the goal is to construct a home environment that sets you up for effortless blood sugar control. When you remove as much friction as possible from healthy eating, it's infinitely easier to stay the course and sidestep common diabetes pitfalls. Here's to stocking your pantry with nourishment!

11. BONUS CHAPTER 3: THE NEXT LEVEL - OPTIMIZING LONGEVITY

If you've made it this far in the book, phenomenal work! That means you've not only successfully reversed your type 2 diabetes through comprehensive lifestyle changes, but you've reclaimed your metabolic health, energy levels, and vitality in the process.

Perhaps you've lost a significant amount of weight, dropped your need for medications entirely, or begun tackling other chronic conditions like high blood pressure or joint pain. No matter how you've leveled up, I want to start by congratulating you. This journey has undoubtedly been immensely challenging, but your perseverance and commitment to prioritizing your well-being is truly inspiring.

So...what's next?

For many, the natural next step is to start pondering how to sustain and build upon these incredible health transformations for the long-term. It's about going from not just surviving, but optimizing for thriving for decades to come through the lens of longevity.

When it comes to cultivating durability of health span (not just life span), continuing to finetune the core pillars of nutrition, exercise, sleep, stress management, and community connection will always remain paramount. But there are also some additional, leading-edge strategies worth exploring in your endless quest for vitality.

In this chapter, I'll share a glimpse into some of the cutting-edge research and emerging practices around extending human health span. From strategic fasting and nutrient cycling to the genetics of aging and hormesis, I'll aim to provide a high-level roadmap for those of you eager to take your wellness optimization to the absolute furthest frontiers of what's possible.

The Longevity Benefits of Fasting

While periods of thoughtful calorie reduction and appetite control were likely part of your initial diabetes reversal protocol, the science of fasting has evolved far beyond just a weight loss tactic. Overwhelming research now points to intermittent, periodic, and prolonged fasts as potent longevity-boosting interventions capable of conferring profound metabolic advantages.

At a basic level, fasting allows your body to intermittently rest from the energy-intensive processes of digesting and metabolizing food. This facilitates a coordinated shift towards various cellular repair, recycling, and rejuvenation pathways that get deprioritized when your body is in a constant fed state.

Specific benefits associated with regular fasting cycles include increased insulin sensitivity, reduced oxidative stress and inflammation, improved cellular adenosine triphosphate (ATP) production, better nutrient sensing and signaling processes, ramped up autophagy (recycling of damaged cells), and potentially even slowed stem cell aging depending on the fasting duration.

For example, shorter intermittent fasts in the 16-24 hour range have been shown to enhance insulin mediated glucose uptake while suppressing insulin resistance - a clear win for sustaining your diabetes remission long-term. Meanwhile, more prolonged multi-day fasts may inhibit a process called IGF-1 downregulation that is closely linked to longevity and tumor suppression.

Of course, any dramatic change in caloric intake should be approached methodically under guidance from a qualified medical and nutrition team. But for many looking to press the advantage on their metabolic rejuvenation, strategic fasting can be an incredible tool.

Nutrient Cycling & Dietary Rhythms

Taking the fasting/feeding approach a step further, a growing body of research supports implementing thoughtful nutrient cycling and dietary rhythms to optimize cellular repair processes and potentially extend healthspan.

The core idea is that by varying influxes of carbohydrates, proteins, and fats in an intelligent, timed manner, you can beneficially stress and upregulate various metabolic pathways in your body. Rather than maintaining a static nutritional state, this dynamic approach taps into a powerful survival mechanism called hormesis - whereby calculated stressors are used to fortify your cells against chronic diseases and environmental exposures.

For example, a brief ketogenic phase focused on healthy fats and low-carb intake can sensitize your body to burning fat as a clean fuel while enhancing autophagy. Then, following that up with bouts of higher protein availability supports muscle growth and regenerative processes like human growth hormone production. Subsequent re-feeds with complex carb sources help reload glycogen stores and facilitate functions like immune regulation.

When properly personalized and cycled, this approach has been shown in animal research to increase mean and maximum life spans while enhancing biomarkers of health like insulin sensitivity and inflammation. Human research is still emerging, but many longevity experts believe nutrient cycling will be a cornerstone of optimizing human vitality in the coming decades.

Of course, this is just the tip of the iceberg when it comes to cutting-edge longevity science. Other intriguing areas of research include:

• Microbiome optimization through pre/probiotic regimens, fecal transplants, etc.

• Epigenetic reprogramming and expressing longevity genes

• Targeted stem cell therapies and organ replacements

• Environmental detoxification routines and interventions like saunas

• Optimizing photobiomodulation and nutrient

absorption via light/magnetic frequencies

• NAD+ IV therapies and other novel nutrients to upregulate sirtuin genes

• Anti-aging pharmacology (rapamycin, metformin, etc.)

The key for all of these emerging areas is to stay curious, continue self-educating, and develop an ecosystem of skilled medical and health professionals who can help guide you responsibly. This is the very frontier of uncovering human potential, so a certain degree of self-experimentation and open-mindedness is required.

Always be prudent about vetting any new products or therapies, start with the most conservative evidence-based protocols, and track your biomarkers to evaluate impact. Longevity science is advancing at a breakneck pace, but discernment is critical.

Building a Community of Lifelong Wellness

Lastly, I want to emphasize that no amount of metabolic tinkering or therapeutic intervention can fully insulate you from the immense importance of nurturing your wealth of social connection and life purpose as you extend your health span.

Having survived your own health crisis, I'm certain you've experienced firsthand how vital a strong community of support and sense of courage/resilience can be. These are not luxuries or nice-to-haves...they are foundational pillars for optimizing your overall quality of life and extending longevity in a truly holistic sense.

So I encourage you to continue deepening the relationships, activities, environments, and sense of meaning that bring you joy, growth, and grounded fulfillment each and every day. Explore ways of giving back, sharing your wisdom, and leaving a positive impact on the world around you. Those sources of intrinsic motivation, awe, and connection to something larger than yourself are potent anti-aging forces.

Seek out and engage with communities of like-minded people also on their own personal wellness journeys. These are the individuals who will inspire you, share resources and insights, hold you accountable, and reinforce your lifestyle commitments long-term. Isolation and lack of emotional nourishment is its own form of metabolic poison.

While the leading-edge technologies and

therapeutic interventions I mentioned above are incredibly promising, always remember that true longevity is about optimizing for quality life years - not just blindly extending life at all costs. It's about cultivating wholeness, meaning, and richness across all aspects of human experience. With intentionality and the right support system in place, you now have the foundations to thrive for an incredibly long time to come.

So keep learning, keep growing, keep asking questions and adjusting your path based on the latest credible science and resources. Most importantly, keep pouring into relationships, cultivating your passions, and reinforcing positive lifestyle anchors like we've discussed throughout this book. You are deeply worthy of experiencing all that an extended human health span has to offer. I'm cheering you on every step of the way!

10. BONUS CHAPTER 2: TRAVEL & DINING OUT TACTICS

One of the most common hurdles people face when making any kind of dramatic lifestyle change is figure out how to sustain those new, healthy habits while traveling or dining out at restaurants. Between irregular schedules, lack of access to a kitchen, social pressures, and the temptation of vacation indulgences, it can feel downright impossible to stick to your diabetes game plan.

Trust me, I've been there! As someone who frequently travels for work and lives in a culinary-obsessed city, those first few months of navigating eating on-the-go were some of the toughest of my journey. I can't tell you how many times I found myself hangry, overwhelmed, and making rash decisions that spiked my blood sugar and drained my willpower.

But over time, through relentless trial-and-error and more than a few hard lessons learned, I developed a toolkit of sustainable strategies for adhering to my diabetes reversal program no matter where my adventures took me. In this chapter, I'm going to share those travel and dining out tactics with you.

The first key is to be proactive about preparing and packing diabetes-friendly snacks and meals whenever possible. Whether you're heading out for a day of sightseeing, have a long road trip ahead, or are about to board a long-haul flight, never leave home without nourishing options to fuel you. Here are some grab-and-go ideas:

• Protein packets or boxes of jerky, turkey sticks, or baked chicken/salmon

• Shelf-stable snacks like nuts, seeds, olives, or prepackaged protein balls

• Fresh veggie sticks and individual nut butter packs for dipping

• String cheese, hard boiled eggs, or precooked shrimp

• Avocados, which make a great addition to any meal

• Keto-friendly protein shakes or powder for mixing with water

Having these staple options on hand allows you to cover your nutritional bases and avoid getting ravenously hungry in compromising situations. I'll often pre-portion items into spill-proof containers so I can easily reach for something while on-the-go.

If I know I'll be somewhere without great access to healthy fare, like an airport or isolated highway, I may also prep full meal options like chef salads with protein and healthy fats, lettuce-wrapped burgers, or cooked veggie portions with seasonings. A little advanced planning can save you from settling for nutrient-void fast food.

For air travel, check if you're allowed to bring your own food through security to have on the plane. Many airlines also offer special meal options you can request ahead of time - just be sure to ask about ingredients and food prep procedures.

Additionally, invest in a portable, insulated cooler bag and ice pack system to ensure perishable items stay fresh in transit. And bring plenty of bottled water to ensure you stay hydrated.

Once you've arrived at your lodging, do a quick nearby grocery run if possible. Stock up on basic supplies like hard-boiled eggs, deli meats, salad greens, avocados, nuts and seeds so you'll always have meal components on hand. Many hotels also offer access to mini-fridges or even basic kitchenettes where you can store and prep foods.

If you have access to a kitchen, even just a basic

one, take advantage of doing basic meal prep like baking protein portions and pre-chopping veggies to streamline food assembly later on.

Now, onto the topic of dining out. This is where that spirit of flexibility I emphasized earlier will really come in handy. The reality is, most restaurant meals are going to be less than ideal for stabilizing blood sugar, even if you order wisely. They tend to be high in refined oils, have hidden sugars, and involve oversized portions.

So my advice is this: make the best choices available to you in the moment, be strategic about portions, and simply don't beat yourself up if you have a less-than-optimal experience. One meal won't derail all your progress if you get right back on track as soon as you can.

That said, there are plenty of tactics for navigating restaurant menus and making smart swaps. Study a menu closely before your visit and have a game plan in place before you start feeling tempted. Things you want to look out for:

• Carb-heavy dishes like pasta, bread baskets, French fries, rice pilaf, etc. Ask for substitutions like a side salad or extra vegetables.

• Sugary condiments, salad dressings, and sauces that are often hidden sources of carbs/sugars. Request these to be served on the side.

• Portion distortion! Don't be afraid to ask for a to-go box right when your meal is served and pack up half before you even start eating.

If ordering apps/starters, stick to lighter veggie or protein-forward options like chicken skewers, baked chicken wings tossed in hot sauce, shrimp cocktails or grilled veggie skewers with a yogurt dip.

For entrees, bun-less burgers with a side salad or bun-free sandwich fillings on a bed of greens are excellent choices. You can also order steaks, baked or grilled seafood and loaded veggie sides like roasted brussels sprouts or grilled asparagus. Just watch out for sugary glazes, breading, and sauces.

If you're the one doing the cooking when traveling, look for local grocery stores or farmer's markets where you can pick up fresh proteins and produce to whip up quick, simple meals. Meal prepping is always easier with a complete kitchen, of course, but I've made do with just a hotel room basics like a mini-fridge, microwave, and electric kettle.

Getting creative with single-serve packs of items like

tuna, guacamole, sliced veggies & boiled eggs from the grocery store deli can allow you to assemble deconstructed meals too.

And for those times when dining options are extremely limited, like at airports or highway rest stops? That's when having a little flexibility and giving yourself grace is key.

Find the best available option that keeps your blood sugar stable and hunger at bay, but don't stress if it's not 100% perfectly aligned with your typical regimen. Maybe you get a basic grilled chicken salad, split a sandwich with a friend giving half the bread away, or piece together a tray of portable items like cheese cubes, nuts and apple slices.

Remember - one suboptimal meal in an otherwise consistent pattern of healthy choices won't derail all your efforts. It's about looking for pockets of opportunity to feed yourself well and making the best choices available to you, not stressing endlessly about perfection. Staying positive and getting right back on track as quickly as possible is what matters most.

Speaking of positivity, one of my favorite travel hacks is scheduling in physical activity that doubles as sightseeing and entertainment! Go for a morning walk or hike in a beautiful new area. Book a bike tour of the city. Take advantage of your hotel gym or rent workout equipment like resistance bands for your room.

Getting your body moving regularly between any travel splurges and jet lag sluggishness pays huge dividends for blood sugar control, energy levels and keeping your mood lifted.

And on that note - don't forget the stress management component of your diabetes plan when you're away from home! Disrupted schedules, unfamiliar environments, lengthy transit periods - all of these factors can have a huge impact on your cortisol levels and, by extension, insulin sensitivity.

Make time for restorative activities before bed like light stretching, breathwork, or meditation even if you're on the road. You'll sleep better, stabilize your circadian rhythms, and offset some of the metabolic impact travel can have. That will pay major dividends when going for that second bun-free burger of the day!

Of course, your specific needs and scenarios will look different from mine, but at the end of the day, it really does come down to maintaining flexibility and making the best choices available in the present moment.

The way I see it, any effort to navigate your food challenges while on the road - even if you miss the mark here and there - is infinitely better than throwing in the towel and going completely off the rails. So give yourself a ton of credit, stay as consistent as you can, and get right back on that horse when you get home.

With each trip and dining out experience, your confidence and travel tactics will only improve. Eventually, it will become second nature to pack your snacks, pre-game the restaurant menu, and prioritize movement no matter where you go.

Embracing travel and restaurants as just another opportunity to flex your problem-solving skills is far more productive than seeing them as obstacles standing between you and success. With the right mindset and consistent effort, adventure and healthy living absolutely can go hand-in-hand.

So explore the world, my friend! Just be prepared with a plan, know your limits, minimize damage where you can, and always keep your eye on the bigger picture reason you started in the first place. Diabetes doesn't have to be your travel restrictor - it just means getting a little more creative along the way.

APPENDIX 1: RECIPES !

Delicious Diabetes-Friendly Recipes

At this point, you have all the knowledge and strategic tools needed to overhaul your nutrition, exercise, sleep, stress management, and more for reversing type 2 diabetes. But putting that into practice through actual meal preparation can sometimes be the biggest challenge.

That's why I wanted to include this dedicated recipe chapter filled with my favorite delicious, nutrient-dense, blood sugar-stabilizing dishes. Consider these your fun exploration into just how satisfying and flavorful eating for sustainable diabetes reversal can be!

From energy-boosting breakfasts and hydrating smoothies to savory meat and veggie-packed main courses, crowd-pleasing sides, and even diabetes-friendly desserts, I've curated an array of simple yet crave-worthy meals the whole family can enjoy.

Many of these recipes can be mixed, matched, and repurposed into portable lunch options or quick-reheat dinners. And they're all crafted with nutrient density at the forefront - featuring healthy fats, lean proteins, low-glycemic carb sources, and loads of fiber to stabilize blood sugar and keep you energized for hours.

So stock up on fresh produce, high-quality proteins, functional pantry staples, and let's get cooking!

Savory Breakfast Patties
Breakfast
Servings: 8 patties

- 1 lb ground breakfast sausage or ground turkey
- 1 cup riced cauliflower or broccoli
- 1/2 cup shredded cheese (cheddar, pepper jack, etc.)
- 1 egg, beaten
- 2 Tbsp everything bagel seasoning or other desired spice blend

1. Preheat oven to 400°F and line a baking sheet with parchment paper.
2. In a bowl, mix together all ingredients until very well combined.
3. Using your hands, form the mixture into 8 equal-sized patties and place on the baking sheet, flattening them slightly.
4. Bake for 15-18 minutes, flipping halfway, until cooked through.
5. Serve alongside a salad or topped with avocado!

Coconut Baked "Oatmeal"
Breakfast
Servings: 4

• 2 eggs
• 1 cup unsweetened almond or coconut milk
• ¼ cup coconut oil, melted
• 1 tsp vanilla extract
• ½ tsp cinnamon
• ¼ tsp nutmeg
• ¼ tsp sea salt
• 1 cup shredded unsweetened coconut
• ¼ cup sliced almonds
• ¼ cup sugar-free maple syrup or monk fruit sweetener

1. Pre-heat oven to 350°F and grease a baking dish with coconut oil.
2. In a bowl, mix together eggs, milk, coconut oil, vanilla, cinnamon, nutmeg, and salt.
3. Fold in the shredded coconut and 2 Tbsp of the sliced almonds.
4. Pour the mixture into the prepared baking dish and top with remaining sliced almonds.
5. Bake for 30-35 minutes until set and lightly browned on top.
6. Drizzle with sugar-free maple syrup before serving.

Summer Shrimp Avocado Salad
Salad
Servings: 4

For the salad:

- 1 lb cooked shrimp, chilled
- 2 avocados, diced
- 1 cup cherry tomatoes, halved
- 1 large cucumber, diced
- ¼ red onion, very thinly sliced
- ½ cup crumbled feta or cotija cheese
- ¼ cup fresh cilantro, chopped

For the dressing:
- 3 Tbsp olive oil
- 2 Tbsp fresh lime juice
- 1 tsp dijon mustard
- 1 garlic clove, minced
- ¼ tsp sea salt
- ¼ tsp black pepper

1. In a large bowl, combine the shrimp, avocado, tomatoes, cucumber, onion, cheese, and cilantro.
2. In a small bowl, whisk together all the dressing ingredients.
3. Pour the dressing over the salad and gently toss to combine.
4. Serve chilled or at room temperature.

Crispy Salmon Cakes with Lemon Dill Sauce
Mains
Servings: 8 cakes

For the salmon cakes:
- 14 oz canned salmon, drained
- 1 egg, beaten

- ¼ cup almond flour
- ½ cup almond meal or finely crushed pork rinds
- ¼ cup diced onion
- 2 Tbsp fresh dill, chopped
- 1 tsp lemon zest
- 1 tsp seafood seasoning or Old Bay
- ¼ tsp salt
- 2 Tbsp olive oil or avocado oil for cooking

For the lemon dill sauce:
- ½ cup plain greek yogurt
- 2 Tbsp olive oil
- 2 Tbsp lemon juice
- 1 Tbsp fresh dill, chopped
- ½ tsp lemon zest
- ⅛ tsp garlic powder
- Pinch of salt

1. In a bowl, mix together all the salmon cake ingredients except the oil until very well combined.
2. Form the mixture into 8 equal patties, firmly pressing to help them hold their shape.
3. Heat the oil in a skillet over medium heat. Cook the salmon cakes for 3-4 minutes per side until browned and crispy.
4. While the cakes cook, make the sauce by mixing all those ingredients together in a bowl.
5. Serve the salmon cakes warm with the lemon dill sauce on the side for dipping or drizzling over top.

Loaded Portobello Mushroom Pizzas

Mains
Servings: 4

- 4 large portobello mushroom caps
- 1 cup shredded mozzarella cheese
- 1 cup finely chopped bell peppers, onions, olives, etc.
- ¼ cup grated parmesan cheese
- 2 garlic cloves, minced
- 1 tsp Italian seasoning
- ¼ tsp salt
- ¼ tsp black pepper
- 2 Tbsp olive oil

1. Remove the stems/gills from the portobello mushroom caps and lightly brush both sides with olive oil.
2. Place the caps on a baking sheet stem side up.
3. In a bowl, mix together the cheeses, veggie toppings, garlic, and seasonings.
4. Divide the mixture evenly between the mushroom caps, pressing to adhere.
5. Bake at 400°F for 12-15 minutes until mushrooms are tender and cheese is melted.
6. Top with marinara sauce, ranch, or any other desired toppings before serving!

Crispy Parmesan Zucchini Fries
Sides
Servings: 4

- 2 medium zucchinis
- 2 eggs
- 2 Tbsp heavy cream or unsweetened almond milk
- 1 cup almond flour
- 1 cup grated parmesan cheese
- 1 tsp Italian seasoning
- ½ tsp salt
- ¼ tsp black pepper
- Olive oil spray

1. Preheat oven to 425°F and line 2 baking sheets with parchment paper.
2. Cut the zucchinis into thick "fry" shaped sticks and pat dry with paper towels.
3. In one bowl, whisk the eggs and cream together.
4. In another bowl, mix the almond flour, parmesan, Italian seasoning, salt, and pepper.
5. Working in batches, dip the zucchini fries first in the egg mixture, then coat thoroughly in the almond flour blend. Place on the baking sheets in a single layer.
6. Mist the fries lightly with olive oil spray.
7. Bake for 20-25 minutes, flipping halfway, until golden brown and crispy.

Fudgy Keto Brownies
Dessert
Servings: 16 brownies

- ½ cup almond butter
- ¼ cup melted cacao butter or coconut oil

- 3 eggs
- ⅓ cup monk fruit sweetener
- ⅓ cup cacao powder
- 1 tsp vanilla extract
- ¼ tsp sea salt
- ¼ cup chopped nuts like pecans or walnuts (optional)

1. Preheat oven to 350°F and grease an 8x8" baking pan.
2. In a bowl, use a hand mixer to blend together the almond butter, melted fat, and eggs until smooth.
3. Add in the sweetener, cacao powder, vanilla, and salt, mixing until fully incorporated and batter is thick and fudgy.
4. Fold in the chopped nuts if using.
5. Pour the batter into the prepared pan and bake for 15-18 minutes until set around the edges but still fudgy in the center.
6. Allow to cool completely before slicing into squares.

I hope these tasty recipes inspire you to keep having fun in the kitchen as you manage your diabetes through a nutrient-dense diet! Remember, sustainable healthy eating is all about discovering new favorite foods and flavors that nourish you from the inside out.

APPENDIX 2: ADDITIVES & SUPPLEMENTS

After long personal research I've made, let's explore some of the most promising nutrients, botanicals, and compounds that have been researched for their potential benefits in regulating blood sugar, enhancing insulin sensitivity, reducing inflammation, and otherwise optimizing metabolic function.

As with any dietary supplement, it's crucial to first consult with your healthcare provider, especially if taking medications, to ensure proper dosing and avoid any adverse interactions. Quality sourcing from reputable brands is also extremely important.

But when used responsibly, these targeted additions to your anti-diabetes toolkit can help amplify and solidify your hard-earned results from diet and lifestyle modification alone.

Alpha-Lipoic Acid

A versatile antioxidant produced naturally in our bodies, alpha-lipoic acid (ALA) has been the subject of extensive research related to its potential for preventing and even reversing diabetic neuropathy and other complications.

ALA has been shown to help reduce oxidative stress, improve glucose uptake into cells, enhance insulin signaling pathways, and protect against protein and mitochondrial damage. It may also reduce biomarkers of inflammation and have a beneficial impact on body weight and lipid profiles.

Look for quality ALA supplements that allow for proper absorption and bioavailability, as it can have a short half-life in the body. Typical doses for diabetes management range from 300-600mg daily, often divided into 2-3 doses with food.

Berberine

Derived from plants like goldenseal and tree turmeric, berberine is an active compound that has garnered significant interest in the diabetes research space for its observed impact on improving insulin resistance and metabolic dysfunction.

Studies have found berberine can help increase insulin receptor expression, support a healthy gut microbiome, reduce glucose production in the liver, and activate metabolic pathways that aid in glucose uptake into cells. It's considered to be as effective as the diabetes drug metformin in some trials.

Berberine is generally very safe and well-tolerated, with typical doses ranging from 500-1500mg daily for therapeutic benefits. People with certain conditions or taking medications may need to avoid berberine, so clear it with your doctor first and start low while assessing your individual response.

Cinnamon & Botanical Extracts

Cinnamon has been used for centuries in Ayurvedic and Traditional Chinese Medicine to help regulate blood sugar, in part due to containing active compounds that can enhance insulin sensitivity. Modern research has provided validation, with cinnamon extracts demonstrating an ability to slow gastric emptying, inhibit digestive enzymes that break down carbs, and improve glucose uptake into cells.

Gymnema sylvestre, bitter melon, fenugreek, ginger, and turmeric are other examples of botanicals and spices that harbor anti-diabetic and metabolic regulating properties. Many of these compounds work through similar pathways as pharmaceuticals like enhancing insulin secretion or inhibiting enzymes involved in carbohydrate metabolism.

When using any concentrated botanical extracts,

be sure to purchase from a reputable supplement brand and follow dosage guidelines. Some may interact with medications or have contraindications for certain individuals. As with all supplements, it's wise to clear new additions with your doctor first.

Chromium and Minerals

The mineral chromium has been shown to play a vital role in amplifying the effects of insulin and improving glucose tolerance. By enhancing the binding of insulin to its receptors, chromium can help facilitate proper glucose uptake into cells and enhance insulin sensitivity.

While overt chromium deficiency is quite rare, subtle insufficiencies are common - especially among populations with poor dietary habits or increased metabolic demands. This is why chromium is often included in glucose control supplements and multivitamin formulas.

Other minerals like zinc, magnesium, and vanadium have also demonstrated favorable impacts on glycemic control and potential benefits for preventing or managing diabetes complications when replenished to proper levels.

High-quality multivitamin/mineral supplements

sourced from whole foods can help ensure you're getting these critical micronutrients. Following dosage guidelines, cycling usage, and testing levels with your doctor can further optimize supplementation.

Omega-3s and Fish Oil

Inflammation and an unhealthy balance of omega fatty acids are thought to be major drivers behind insulin resistance and the cascade towards type 2 diabetes. This is where anti-inflammatory omega-3s from fish oil, krill oil, or plant sources like algae can provide metabolic benefits.

Research indicates that increasing omega-3 intake, particularly EPA and DHA found in marine sources, can enhance insulin sensitivity, support healthy triglyceride levels, reduce oxidative stress, and even preserve insulin-producing beta cell function in some cases.

Standard fish oil doses of 1-4 grams per day of an omega-3 concentrate containing both EPA and DHA have been used effectively in diabetic populations. As with any supplement, choose a high-quality source tested for purity and freshness.

Fiber Additives

We know that one of the core nutritional pillars of diabetes prevention and management is increasing your intake of fiber-rich foods like leafy greens, berries, nuts, and seeds. But sometimes, even the most health-conscious individual can use a little extra boost in the fiber department.

This is where soluble and insoluble fiber supplements like psyllium husk, glucomannan, acacia fiber, and resistant starches can provide valuable support. These functional fibers help slow the absorption of glucose into the bloodstream, improve feelings of satiety, and nourish your beneficial gut microbes.

When taking supplemental fibers, it's important to start slowly and ramp up dosages gradually while drinking plenty of water to avoid gastrointestinal discomfort. Look for products free of unnecessary binders and fillers as well.

This is just a highlight reel of some of the most promising nutrients, botanicals, and compounds that emerging research is uncovering for use in diabetes management protocols. The science is rapidly evolving, but the potential is incredibly exciting.

As always, the core tenets of an anti-inflammatory,

low-glycemic, whole foods based diet is the foundation. But when used responsibly under your doctor's guidance, judicious supplementation can add another layer of metabolic support and protection against complications.

So stay curious, keep researching, and don't be afraid to have open, informed conversations with your healthcare team about supplement quality, proper dosing, and any unique factors in your case. An integrated, personalized multi-therapy approach may be your path toward optimal results!

ABOUT THE AUTHOR

James S. Andersen

James "The Diabetes Disruptor" Andersen is on a mission to rewrite the narrative around type 2 diabetes. As a regular guy - a computer programmer with a wife, three kids, and two cats - he refused to resign himself to the grim prognosis of a chronic, progressive disease. Through meticulous research, experimentation, and an unwavering commitment to lifestyle transformation, James was able to completely reverse his type 2 diabetes in a matter of months - no more medications, painful injections, or compromise of quality of life. In his debut book, he pulls back the curtain on the strategies and mindset shifts that allowed him to regain control of his metabolic health, guiding readers through the same holistic approach he used to systematically dismantle the root causes of his insulin resistance.